Caring for Someone with PTSD:

A practical guide to loving your partner after trauma

Barbara V. Tran, Ph.D.

All rights reserved. No part of this publication may be reproduced, distributed, or transmitted in any form or by any means, including photocopying, recording, or other electronic or mechanical methods, without the prior written permission of the publisher, except in the case of brief quotations embodied in critical reviews and certain other noncommercial uses permitted by copyright law.

Copyright © (Barbara V. Tran, Ph.D.), (2022).

Table of Contents

Chapter 1

[Chapter 2](#)

[Chapter 3](#)

[Chapter 4](#)

[Chapter 5](#)

[Chapter 6](#)

Chapter 1

What is PTSD and What It isn't?

What is Posttraumatic Stress Disorder (PTSD)?

Posttraumatic stress disorder (PTSD) is a mental illness that may emerge in persons who have experienced or seen a traumatic incident, sequence of events, or set of circumstances. It is a mental health disorder that's caused by a horrific incident - either experiencing it or seeing it. Symptoms may include flashbacks, nightmares, and acute anxiety, as well as uncontrolled thoughts about the incident.

A person may feel this as emotionally or physically hurtful or life-threatening and may damage mental, bodily, social, and/or spiritual well-being. Examples include natural catastrophes, major accidents, terrorist attacks, war/combat, rape/sexual assault, historical trauma, intimate relationship abuse, and bullying.

PTSD has been called by various names in the past, such as "shell shock" during the years of World War I and "battle fatigue" following World War II, but PTSD does not simply happen to combat veterans. PTSD may occur in all individuals, of any race, country, or culture, and at any age. PTSD affects around 3.5 percent of U.S. adults every year.

The lifetime prevalence of PTSD among teenagers aged 13 -18 is 8%. An estimated one in 11 persons will be diagnosed with PTSD in their lifetime. Women are twice as likely as males to experience PTSD. Three ethnic groups – U.S. Latinos, African Americans, and Native Americans/Alaska Natives – are disproportionately afflicted and have greater rates of PTSD than non-Latino whites.

People with PTSD have powerful, distressing thoughts and sensations relating to their experience that remain long after the traumatic event has finished. They may re-experience the event through flashbacks or nightmares; they may feel sadness, fear, or anger; and they may feel detached or distanced from other people. People with PTSD may avoid situations or people that remind them of the traumatic event, and they may have strong negative reactions to something as normal as a loud noise or an accidental touch.

A diagnosis of PTSD requires exposure to an upsetting traumatic event. Exposure includes directly experiencing an event, watching a traumatic event happening to others, or learning that a horrific incident happened to a close family member or friend. It can also occur as a result of repeated exposure to horrible details of trauma such as police officers being exposed to details of child abuse cases.

What's traumatic to you might not be for someone else, though. In this way, trauma is a private process that's unique to each individual. What counts is how you feel and how you live through that experience.

Some individuals get PTSD after encountering a frightening experience. Other individuals can get the syndrome by watching this awful incident from a distance.

For example, if you've just heard of a family tragedy or if you have work where you routinely observe abuse situations, you can acquire PTSD.

The circumstances leading up to a diagnosis may also impact the sorts of symptoms you'll encounter.

PTSD as the consequence of sexual assault, for example, may show differently than PTSD due to a vehicle accident or military service.

The triggers of PTSD could also make a difference in how you approach your relationships if you have the disorder. In the same way, not everyone will acquire PTSD when exposed to the same experiences, not everyone will suffer the same PTSD symptoms or obstacles that come with it.

Feeling or behaving this way isn't anything to feel bad about. These are normal reactions to trauma that may be handled and improved with time.

Most individuals who have experienced traumatic circumstances may have some difficulties adapting and coping, but with time and proper self-care, they generally get better. If the symptoms develop worse, linger for months or even years, and interfere with your day-to-day functioning, you may have PTSD.

Getting appropriate therapy after PTSD symptoms start might be crucial to lessen symptoms and enhance function.

Symptoms and Diagnosis

Post-traumatic stress disorder symptoms may start within one month of a traumatic event, but sometimes symptoms may not appear until years after the event. These symptoms cause significant problems in social or work situations and in relationships. They can also interfere with your ability to go about your normal daily tasks.

Symptoms of PTSD can vary over time or vary from person to person. They fall into the following four categories. Specific symptoms can vary in severity.

Intrusion: Intrusive thoughts such as repeated, involuntary memories; distressing dreams; or flashbacks of the traumatic event. Flashbacks may be so vivid that people feel they are reliving the traumatic experience or seeing it before their eyes.

Avoidance: Avoiding reminders of the traumatic event may include avoiding people, places, activities, objects, and situations that may trigger distressing memories. People may try to avoid remembering or thinking about the traumatic event. They may resist talking about what happened or how they feel about it.

Alterations in cognition and mood: Inability to remember important aspects of the traumatic event, negative thoughts and feelings leading to ongoing and distorted beliefs about oneself or others (e.g., "I am bad," "No one can be trusted"); distorted thoughts about the cause or consequences of the event leading to wrongly blaming self or other; ongoing fear, horror, anger, guilt or shame; much less interest in activities previously enjoyed; feeling detached or estranged from others; or being unable to experience positive emotions (a void of happiness or satisfaction).

Alterations in arousal and reactivity: Arousal and reactive symptoms may include being irritable and having angry outbursts; behaving recklessly or in a self-destructive way; being overly watchful of one's surroundings in a suspecting way; being easily startled, or having problems concentrating or sleeping.

Many people who are exposed to a traumatic event experience symptoms similar to those described above in the days following the event. For a person to be diagnosed with PTSD, however, symptoms must last for more than a month and must cause significant distress or problems in the individual's daily functioning.

Many individuals develop symptoms within three months of the trauma, but symptoms may appear later and often persist for months and sometimes years. PTSD often occurs with other related conditions, such as depression, substance use, memory problems, and other physical and mental health problems.

PTSD symptoms can vary in intensity over time. You may have more PTSD symptoms when you're stressed in general, or when you come across reminders of what you went through. For example, you may hear a car backfire and relive combat experiences. Or you may see a report on the news about a sexual assault and feel overcome by memories of your own assault.

Treatment

It is important to note that not everyone who experiences trauma develops PTSD, and not everyone who develops PTSD requires psychiatric treatment.

For some people, symptoms of PTSD subside or disappear over time. Others get better with the help of their support system (family, friends, or clergy). But many people with PTSD need professional treatment to recover from psychological distress that can be intense and disabling.

It is important to remember that trauma may lead to severe distress. That distress is not the individual's fault, and PTSD is treatable. The earlier a person gets treatment, the better chance of recovery.

PTSD is a complex mental health condition. Effective treatment may include making lifestyle changes, getting family support, seeking therapy, or taking medication.

Some possible treatments for PTSD include:

Therapy: The American Psychological Association recommends cognitive behavioral therapy, cognitive processing therapy, cognitive therapy, and prolonged exposure therapy.

Medication: Some medications may help with PTSD symptoms. These include antidepressants, anti anxiety medications, and, in some cases, sleeping medications.

Couples counseling: Relationship counseling will not cure PTSD, but it may help with relationship problems, including those that stem from PTSD. A 2015 study, for example, suggests using emotionally focused therapy for couples. This approach focuses on nurturing the couple's attachments and providing mutual support.

Education: Learning as much as possible about PTSD can help both partners understand the diagnosis, separate relationship problems from PTSD-related issues, and identify effective treatment strategies.

Lifestyle changes: People with PTSD sometimes find symptom relief from self-management strategies such as meditating, exercising, joining a support group, and talking to loved ones.

Psychiatrists and other mental health professionals use various effective (research-proven) methods to help people recover from PTSD. Both talk therapy (psychotherapy) and medication provide effective evidence-based treatments for PTSD.

When to visit a doctor

- If you experience worrisome thoughts and emotions about a traumatic occurrence for more than a month, if they're serious, or if you feel you're having difficulties bringing your life back under control, speak to your doctor or a mental health expert. Undergoing therapy as soon as possible will help avoid PTSD symptoms from getting worse.
- If you experience suicidal thoughts

- If you or someone you know has suicidal thoughts, seek assistance right immediately.
- Reach out to a close friend or loved one.
- Contact a clergyman, a spiritual leader, or someone in your religious group.
- Make an appointment with your doctor or mental health professional.

When to receive emergency help

- If you fear you may injure yourself or attempt suicide, contact 911 or your local emergency number immediately.
- If you know someone who's at risk of trying suicide or has made a suicide attempt, make sure someone remains with that person to keep him or her safe. Call 911 or your local emergency number immediately. Or, if you can do so safely, transport the individual to the closest hospital emergency department.

Causes

You may acquire post-traumatic stress disorder when you go through, observe or learn about an incident involving real or threatened death, severe injury, or sexual violation.

Doctors aren't clear why certain individuals suffer from PTSD. As with other mental health disorders, PTSD is probably caused by a complicated combination of:

- Stressful situations, including the number and degree of a trauma you've gone through in your life
- Inherited mental health concerns, such as a family history of anxiety and depression
- Inherited characteristics of your personality — commonly termed your temperament
- The way your brain manages the chemicals and hormones your body produces in reaction to stress

Risk factors

People of all ages may develop post-traumatic stress disorder. However, several variables may make you more susceptible to acquiring PTSD following a distressing incident, such as:

- Experiencing intense or long-lasting trauma
- Having experienced other trauma earlier in life, such as childhood abuse
- Having a job that increases your risk of being exposed to traumatic events, such as military personnel and first responders
- Having other mental health problems, such as anxiety or depression
- Having problems with substance misuse, such as excess drinking or drug use
- Lacking a good support system of family and friends
- Having biological relations with mental health disorders, particularly anxiety or depression

Complications

Post-traumatic stress disorder may impact your entire life — your career, your relationships, your health, and your pleasure in ordinary activities.

Having PTSD may also raise your chance of other mental health disorders, such as:

- Depression and anxiety
- Issues with drugs or alcohol use
- Eating disorders
- Suicidal thoughts and acts

Prevention

After surviving a terrible experience, many individuals exhibit PTSD-like symptoms at first, such as being unable to stop thinking about what's occurred. Fear, anxiety, rage, melancholy, guilt – these are normal responses to trauma.

However, the majority of persons exposed to trauma do not acquire long-term post-traumatic stress disorder.

Getting timely help and support may hinder stress reactions from getting worse and developing into PTSD. This may mean turning to family and friends who will listen and offer comfort. It may mean seeking out a mental health professional for a brief course of therapy. Some people may also find it helpful to turn to their faith community.

Support from others also may help prevent you from turning to unhealthy coping methods, such as misuse of alcohol or drugs.

Common myths about PTSD

Here are five common myths people believe about PTSD — and why they aren't true.

1. Military veterans are the only ones who get PTSD

Though factually false, the belief that PTSD affects only military veterans who've experienced war-related trauma is understandable. After all, it was just in 1980 — five years after the Vietnam War ended — that the American Psychiatric Association added PTSD to its Diagnostic and Statistical Manual of Mental Disorders (then in its third edition).

Of course, the symptoms linked with the disorder have always existed for those who suffered following a traumatic experience, but this was the first group to be given a diagnosis of PTSD.

This misperception may be hazardous. A person who has suffered trauma and is displaying signs of PTSD may not be prompted to seek out a diagnosis since he or she hasn't been in the military and doesn't identify PTSD with other types of trauma.

In reality, PTSD may impact individuals who have gone through a sexual assault, people who have endured vehicle accidents and terrorist attacks, and those who have suffered from domestic violence and lived through national catastrophes.

Also contrary to common assumption, a person doesn't have to suffer a life-threatening incident to get PTSD. For instance, finding that a loved one endured trauma might lead to PTSD.

2. PTSD is a chronic condition that can't be treated effectively

Another misunderstanding regarding PTSD is that this mental disease can't be cured. This is certifiably untrue. There are various therapies available for those who are struggling with the impacts of a traumatic incident. The National Institute for Mental Health gives a summary of some of these therapy methods.

Psychotherapy: It is also known as "talk therapy." This entails conversing with a mental health expert, and it might take place one-on-one with a psychiatrist or psychologist or in a group environment. You could employ relaxation and anger-management techniques to cope with assessing your response to the event. A therapist may also assist you with sleep, food, and exercise recommendations to help you modify your day-to-day living patterns.

Exposure Therapy: This style of psychotherapy includes addressing and controlling your anxieties. This implies that a therapist might expose you to your triggers (items that remind you of your trauma) by employing mental images of the trauma or having you visit the scene of a traumatic incident.

Cognitive Processing: This is another sort of psychotherapy that seeks to help you make sense of terrible memories related to your trauma. You may feel guilt or shame over your trauma, and a therapist would help you reevaluate why you feel this way.

Medications: Antidepressants are the most popular medications used to assist PTSD. These drugs might help minimize your emotions of melancholy, anger, and anxiety. They could be recommended in addition to your psychotherapy sessions. Always ask your physician or healthcare provider for the drugs and prescriptions that make the most sense for treating your symptoms.

3. Everyone who has PTSD is prone to violent behavior

While related to PTSD, violence is not a prevalent sign of the mental condition.

One of the greatest fallacies out there is that a person with PTSD is a ticking time bomb ready to blow. There is this idea that all individuals who suffer from PTSD are unstable. Now, it is true that persons with PTSD are prone to be irritable, but PTSD has a broad spectrum of symptoms and this concept that everyone who has PTSD is going to burst is a mischaracterization.

Rather, those afflicted by PTSD tend to display avoidance behaviors, causing them to be socially isolated and prone to being terrified of meeting anything that may possibly evoke memories of their experiences.

The U.S. Department of Veterans Affairs lists one research that looked at violent conduct among jailed veterans. At the time, the veteran population in the United States was 24 million, and out of this amount, there were 140,000 veterans in jail. Of that population, nearly 21,000 had been convicted of murder. This made up less than 1/10 of 1 percent for the whole veteran community at large, suggesting that violence was an aberration in this specific demographic at that time.

4. If trauma happened long ago, you get over it automatically

PTSD may be triggered years after a person encounters trauma. Symptoms normally show up approximately three months after a stressful occurrence, but you might acquire the illness years, even decades, later.

That may be particularly true when it comes to trauma encountered at a young age. Someone might encounter a childhood trauma and never process it until much later. It might be something they never spoke about and then something occurs throughout their maturity to awaken that memory and it could start increasing symptoms of PTSD. This is typically evident in those who underwent childhood physical or sexual abuse. They could have repressed memories of this trauma and then get aroused later on when they are grownups.

Many Vietnam veterans endured their trauma approximately 50 years ago yet are influenced by trigger events for their PTSD decades later.

5. Coping with PTSD is a sign of weakness

One disturbing lie is the assumption that persons who suffer from PTSD are "weak."

A lot of times people can think, 'Oh, that person who has PTSD is weak, they're readily vulnerable to trauma.'

It is not a weakness and it isn't something that individuals 'should simply get over,' as they can be advised by misguided others. In reality, it's the reverse; it's very daring when individuals come out to seek therapy and aid and are open to sharing and exploring their trauma.

How to Tell If You Have Normal Post-Traumatic Stress or PTSD

Both mental health issues may emerge after you've suffered trauma, but there's a major difference between them.

When something horrific happens—you abruptly lose a loved one, get into a car disaster, or witness a terrorist attack—normal it's to be tremendously upset and perhaps feel physically unwell. Your "fight or flight" reaction kicks in, overwhelming your body with stress chemicals that make you restless and on edge. You can have dreams about the occurrence or break down in tears when you see or hear anything that reminds you of it.

That's post-traumatic stress (PTS), and it's not a disorder—at least not yet.

PTS is considered a natural response to stress and not a mental disease. It's common and generally resolves on its own. Say you nearly missed an accident on a route notorious for being deadly. You may avoid the road and adjust your path. You may even feel worried about driving along a similar route. You may subsequently dream about the accident you dodged. But after a few days, these ideas diminish and gradually dissipate.

Most of the time, that's precisely what happens: A distressing incident happens, and it shakes you up, but after a few days or weeks, it's no longer a serious concern. No therapy is essential, however, anything that helps you relax—deep breathing, yoga, painting, exercise—might help you feel better and speed the process along.

However, post-traumatic stress disorder (PTSD) is distinct.

PTSD doesn't go away so soon, and your typical de-stressing tactics aren't adequate to help you feel better. Instead, you stay highly apprehensive, repeat the occurrence over and over in your mind, avoid anything that can trigger your memories of it, and remain on high alert for danger.

If you experience these symptoms for at least one month and they're serious enough that they interfere with your regular life, then you could have PTSD. The symptoms might start immediately after a tragedy, or they could first occur months or years later, according to the PTSD Alliance, a national advocacy group.

One frequent misperception is that PTSD exclusively occurs in military veterans. While it's true that the illness is frequent among soldiers—up to 30% of those in active conflict zones eventually get it—also it's pretty common in the general population. An estimated 8% of all Americans have PTSD, and women are twice as likely as men to be impacted by this anxiety disease. It may occur in everyone exposed to a horrific, traumatic experience, regardless of age or background.

Is it PTSD?

Only a skilled mental health specialist can diagnose PTSD, and the length of your symptoms is only half of the story. The American Mental Association describes it as a psychiatric disease that may emerge in persons who have encountered or seen a traumatic event such as a natural catastrophe, a major accident, a terrorist attack, war/combat, rape, or other violent personal assault.

In order to be diagnosed with OCD, a person must experience extended unsettling thoughts that interfere with their regular everyday routines. They may experience highly vivid flashbacks that throw them right back into the horrific situation as if it is occurring again and again.

Intense dreams are quite prevalent, as is the inclination to isolate from friends and family. Someone with PTSD will be very avoidant of undertaking any activity that may even remind them of the trauma they endured. They also may be activated by loud noises, specific odors, sounds, or other recollections. They frequently report they feel jumpy and may look quite shocked at the least contact.

If you're diagnosed with PTSD, treatment, and medication will likely be in order.

There are various sorts of treatments that you may attempt, but extended exposure therapy and cognitive processing therapy are the most extensively utilized and beneficial. Prolonged exposure treatment entails working closely with a specialist to revisit the event and your response to it until you learn to connect it with less anguish.

Cognitive processing therapy is a sort of cognitive behavioral therapy aimed to question your views about the trauma and associated triggers so you may enhance your day-to-day functioning.

Most patients need at least 12 to 15 weeks of treatment to overcome PTSD, although occasionally the disease stays chronic. That implies you may require some form of therapy for the rest of your life in order to feel your best.

Chapter 2

Effect of PTSD on Relationships

Trauma survivors with PTSD may have problems with their intimate family connections or friendships. The symptoms of PTSD may create issues with trust, connection, communication, and problem resolution. These difficulties may impact the way the survivor behaves with others. In turn, the way a loved one reacts to him or her influences the trauma survivor. A cyclical pattern may emerge that may occasionally hurt relationships.

The symptoms of post-traumatic stress disorder (PTSD) may make any relationship challenging. It is challenging for many persons with PTSD to connect to other people in a healthy manner when they have issues with trust, intimacy, and other crucial components of relationships. However, social support may aid persons with PTSD, and professional therapy can steer them toward stronger connections.

How trauma survivors might react

In the early weeks and months after a trauma, survivors may feel angry, disconnected, tense, or frightened in their relationships. In time, most are able to recover their earlier degree of intimacy in relationships. Yet the 5% to 10% of survivors who acquire PTSD may have persistent interpersonal troubles.

Survivors with PTSD may feel alienated from others and feel numb. They may have less interest in social or sexual activities. Because survivors feel irritated, on guard, jumpy, concerned, or frightened, they may not be able to relax or be intimate. They may also sense a heightened urge to defend their loved ones. They may come out as uptight or demanding.

The trauma survivor may frequently experience trauma memories or flashbacks. He or she could go to considerable efforts to prevent such recollections.

Survivors may avoid any behavior that might trigger a recollection. If the survivor has difficulties sleeping or has nightmares, both the survivor and partner may not be able to get adequate rest. This may make sleeping together tougher.

Survivors typically battle with extreme anger and urge. In an attempt to repress hostile sentiments and acts, they may shun proximity. They may push away or find fault with loved ones and friends. Also, alcohol and drug issues, which might be an effort to deal with PTSD, can shatter relationships and friendships. Verbal or physical aggression might erupt.

In other circumstances, survivors may rely too much on their partners, family members, and friends. This might also include support personnel such as health care professionals or therapists.

Dealing with these symptoms might take up a lot of the survivor's focus. He or she may not be able to concentrate on the relationship. It may be challenging to listen intently and make choices jointly with someone else. Partners may begin to believe that communicating together and functioning as a team is not feasible.

How loved ones might react

Partners, friends, or family members may feel wounded, cut off, or depressed because the survivor has not been able to get over the experience. Loved ones may become resentful or aloof from the survivor. They may feel pushed, anxious, and controlled.

The survivor's symptoms might make a loved one feel that he or she is living in a war zone or under continual fear of harm. Living with someone who has PTSD may often cause the spouse to experience some of the same sentiments of having gone through trauma.

In conclusion, a person who has undergone trauma may have some typical responses. These responses influence the individuals around the survivor. Family, friends, and others then respond to how the survivor is acting. This in turn comes back to impact the individual who went through the trauma.

Do all trauma survivors have relationship problems?

Many trauma survivors do not acquire PTSD. Also, many persons with PTSD do not have interpersonal issues. People with PTSD may build and maintain healthy connections by:

- Building a personal support network to assist deal with PTSD while working on family and friend connections
- Sharing sentiments honestly and freely, with respect and compassion
- Building abilities at problem-solving and engaging with others
- Including methods to play, be creative, relax, and appreciate others

What can be done to help someone who has PTSD?

Relations with others are particularly crucial for trauma survivors. Social support is one of the strongest ways to guard against developing PTSD. Relationships may counter the emotions of being alone.

Relationships may also boost the survivor's self-esteem. This may help alleviate sadness and guilt. A connection might also provide the survivor with a means to assist someone else. Helping others might minimize emotions of failure or feeling cut off from others. Lastly, relationships are a source of help while dealing with stress.

If you need to seek professional treatment, try to identify a therapist who has experience in treating PTSD as well as dealing with couples or families.

Many therapeutic options may be beneficial for coping with relationship troubles. Options include:

- One-to-one and group counseling
- Anger and stress management
- Assertiveness training
- Couples counseling
- Family education courses
- Family therapy

How does PTSD affect relationships?

You care about people close to you, but PTSD may sometimes make it difficult for you to engage with them. You could say things you don't mean, or feel unable to relax and be personal.

In reaction, others around you may retreat or become unreceptive, establishing a loop in the connection that may be tough to escape.

But living with PTSD doesn't mean you have to give up on relationships with other people.

It's feasible to treat symptoms of PTSD to enhance your social skills and relationships. In turn, individuals around you may also understand what living with PTSD entails and how to best assist your recovery process.

You didn't choose to get PTSD or to have it influence your relationships. But PTSD symptoms may alter the way you interact with people, even if you're not always conscious of it.

For instance, PTSD could make it hard to communicate, which might make you feel nervous about relationship-building events.

Both personal and professional relationships may be damaged by PTSD. A person may help a partner with PTSD by encouraging them to speak about their emotions when they feel comfortable.

Research reveals a correlation between PTSD and interpersonal troubles. PTSD may bring significant problems to relationships in numerous ways, including:

- feeling a lack of emotional regulation
- losing interest in family activities
- having no interest in sexual activities
- retraumatization during sexual engagement
- feeling increasingly dependent on a partner
- experiencing excess anger, which may come out as being aloof, critical, or abusive
- having a diminished capacity to problem solve
- making the spouse without PTSD feel as if they have to be a caregiver
- reducing the support that couples receive from family members who do not comprehend the trauma or recognize the severity of PTSD

Some persons with PTSD may not seek therapy or acquire the appropriate diagnosis. Therefore, couples should be cognizant that PTSD may impair a relationship even when neither individual has an official diagnosis.

A 2013 research on veterans revealed a correlation between PTSD and relationships with increased anger and psychological abuse, as well as less acceptance and humor, in both veterans and their romantic partners.

Previous research from 2010 on military veterans with PTSD revealed more parental disputes, less confidence in their relationships, more negative communication, and poorer marital satisfaction.

According to the U.S. Department of Veterans Affairs, around 5 to 10% of persons with PTSD could have issues in their relationships involving:

1. Intimacy

Intimacy denotes a connection within a relationship that might be emotional or sexual – and frequently both. This involves talking about your feelings and reacting to the other person's needs.

Intimacy in relationships may be impacted when you live with specific symptoms of PTSD, such as:

- lack of interest in interesting activities
- bad self-image
- feelings disconnected from others, or a difficulty to emotionally connect

Someone with PTSD could feel the urge to be intimate with their spouse but find themselves scared or unable to create such a connection.

2. Sexual interest

The way PTSD impacts your sex life and desire might be difficult. If and how it affects you might also depend on the sort of event that prompted PTSD in the first place.

In circumstances of sexual abuse or trauma, sex could become the top thing on your avoidance list.

This form of trauma could also make it tough to trust a partner or feel secure in a physically intimate scenario. This is a normal response to adversity.

In other circumstances, research shows that trauma could result in hypersexuality. While a controversial issue, hypersexuality is commonly characterized as someone exhibiting obsessive sexual habits that are difficult to control.

Other symptoms of PTSD could also impair your sex life, like:

- bad self-image
- slack of sleep
- slow sex drive
- feeling detached
- hypervigilance that makes resting difficult
- loss of interest in enjoying enjoyable activities

This can be the reason why even if you love your partner so much, you nevertheless feel uninterested or afraid about physical closeness with them.

3. Communication

Communication is crucial in any relationship. When it becomes a struggle for you, it could impair your connection with loved ones.

PTSD symptoms might include irritation and emotional outbursts. You could then react to others in a manner they don't understand, fear, or dislike.

Other symptoms — such as problem-solving issues — could also impact how you cope with disagreements.

Even the slightest talk could make you feel really uncomfortable and overwhelmed, which might get in the way of you expressing yourself correctly.

You could also have times when you don't want to communicate at all, and you simply want to be left alone. Not expressing how you feel could become an obstacle to establishing connections.

4. Avoidance

If you're avoiding certain triggers, you may also want to forgo particular social situations or avoid discussing unpleasant issues.

This is because while you live with PTSD, certain events, people, or activities may remind you of the incident that sparked your illness.

While this is common with trauma, it may make sustaining connections difficult if you don't want to do certain things and can't explain why.

5. Attachment

Being able to connect with people emotionally is vital in relationships. When you live with PTSD, you could feel distant from circumstances, others, and sometimes even yourself. This separation might translate into pushing others away or not being emotionally receptive.

On the other hand, your PTSD symptoms can have you feeling the opposite.

You might have a heightened urge to be taken care of or to protect others. You could then act in demanding, suffocating, or reliant ways that might overwhelm others.

How to support a spouse with PTSD

PTSD is a significant medical condition. It is crucial for a partner to realize that it is not a choice and not something that another person can fix. Strong connections are vital for everyone's well-being, and poor relationships may make recovery from PTSD more difficult.

Supporting a partner may give them the environment they need to seek recovery while expressing reassurance might remind them that someone loves them and is there for them.

To help a spouse with PTSD, a person can:

- Avoid blaming them for their symptoms, diminishing the gravity of their trauma, and asking them to "snap out of it."
- Encourage them to get therapy and offer to assist them to do so.
- If the spouse has thoughts of suicide, consult with a therapist to build a suicide prevention strategy. Remove any weapons from the home.
- Encourage the loved one to speak about their emotions if they wish, but avoid pressing them to do so.
- Do not tell someone how to feel or provide unwanted advice.
- Recognize the influence of PTSD on the relationship, but do not blame all of its issues on PTSD.
- Identify the other person's triggers and attempt to reduce their exposure to them. For example, if loud sounds or voices are a trigger, avoid leaving the television on.
- Talk about methods to reduce the influence of PTSD on the relationship. For example, some persons with PTSD may

dread abandonment, so making threats to leave may increase their symptoms and make the conflict worse.
- Be attentive and compassionate to their feelings. Offer comfort and warmth, particularly during flashbacks or moments of severe anxiety.
- Know that it is OK to walk away. Romantic partners and other loved ones are not qualified therapists and are not ready to cope with all of the challenges that PTSD may bring. It is crucial for a spouse to preserve their own emotions in times that seem overwhelming or extremely tough.

Some persons with PTSD become abusive. While much of the research on PTSD and domestic partner violence has focused on war veterans, it is uncertain if abusive conduct is the outcome of PTSD in general or combat-related PTSD in particular.

People whose spouses abuse them should seek protection as soon as possible. This may entail abandoning the relationship.

Although couples therapy may assist with marital issues, most counselors advise avoiding treatment when there is domestic abuse. It is not safe to stay with an abusive spouse.

A therapist or other healthcare expert may build a strategy to assist a couple to deal with trauma and establish new methods of articulating their needs in a relationship.

Ways to improve relationships

The first step in avoiding PTSD from influencing relationships badly is to become aware of the symptoms and causes. Some persons who struggle with post-traumatic stress may utilize dangerous coping techniques such as alcohol addiction or self-harm.

Whether you're straightforward or honest with your loved ones, they might also feel sorrow that they can't help you or make it easier which can cause an end to romantic partnerships.

Many of the symptoms of post-traumatic stress disorder (PTSD) might interfere with establishing a good relationship. The four forms of symptoms include experiencing flashbacks or dreams about the trauma, avoiding circumstances connected with the trauma, feeling uneasy or irritated, and having elevated negative thoughts and emotions.

These symptom categories might express themselves in a number of ways. For instance, a sound or event can abruptly trigger a flashback, and the person with PTSD might cease wanting to spend time with loved ones, feel low a lot, have difficulties trusting others, avoid particular areas, and suddenly get furious.

These types of responses may make partnerships more challenging on a daily basis. However, relationships may assist individuals with their

PTSD symptoms, in addition to the ongoing support and direction of professional therapy.

Even though relationships may be challenging for someone with PTSD, social support can be useful by raising self-esteem, offering closeness, placing a focus on others, and helping the individual manage stress.

People with PTSD may work on strengthening their relationships by having an empathetic support system, working on interpersonal skills, being honest about their emotions, and finding methods to relax and loosen up with other people.

Their loved ones may aid themselves and the person with PTSD by:

- Not perceiving or treating the individual like he or she has a permanent handicap
- Not being excessively empathetic
- Not feeling responsible for the issue or the healing

- Learning about symptoms and that they're not the person's responsibility
- Engaging in social situations without the loved one
- Working on healthy coping methods
- Making healthy lifestyle adjustments and participating in self-care
- Trying to prevent being codependent

Also, professional therapy may aid persons with PTSD and their loved ones. Both sides may depend on individual, group, couple, and family therapy to assist work through their symptoms and relationship issues. The individual with PTSD may require more rigorous therapy delivered via an inpatient facility.

The symptoms that accompany post-traumatic stress disorder may challenge any relationship. However, identifying the signs and getting therapy may help both parties maintain a better relationship. Social support may improve a person's PTSD, thus focusing on the connection can assist everyone involved.

Trouble areas for people with PTSD

Because trauma survivors typically resist impulsive behavior and extreme rage, personal relationships may seem like minefields. We've all been in the situation of responding too soon and snapping at a spouse; for someone with PTSD, this is a heightened danger.

The "solution" they typically select is avoiding contact and pushing loved ones away "for their own good." They could also find fault with everything their friends and loved ones do, for the same reason. Drug and alcohol addiction is another sanctuary for victims.

Unfortunately, in certain situations, mental abuse or even physical violence may happen. Remember, if it does, there is never any reason for aggressive action. Nevertheless, PTSD patients will undoubtedly feel bad about their lack of control and may recognize that they have a problem if they are challenged by friends and family about their conduct. However, if you have been the object of abuse, don't take risks and address a trauma sufferer yourself. Get to safety instead.

In other cases, survivors could become excessively reliant upon family members, their spouses, their friends, or even therapists or healthcare professionals. Trained healthcare specialists and mental health professionals know how to handle and help cope with this, but if you're a friend or family member, you may not. If a therapist or doctor is in the picture, let them know what's going on, and seek out assistance from others so you're not fighting on your own.

Partners, family members, and acquaintances of persons with PTSD typically have a hard time dealing with all of this. They could feel alone, despondent, or wounded since they are unable to assist the victim move over the trauma, and they might not know where to turn. They could also feel restricted and tight and become aloof or even furious with the individual suffering from PTSD. Some survivors have a knack for making the people around them feel like they too are living in a battle zone.

Coping with PTSD in a relationship

Coping with PTSD in a relationship isn't easy, but there are methods to strive toward happier, healthier relationships as you recover from traumatic situations. People with PTSD may form and keep good relationships by working on the following things:

- Develop a network of personal support to aid in the coping process with PTSD and help create deeper ties with friends and family
- Learn to communicate your feelings—even those that concern or fear you—openly and honestly, always with compassion and respect

- Build communication, problem-solving, and connection skills by engaging with people
- Practice being creative, fun, relaxing, and enjoying your time, both alone and with others

How can you obtain assistance performing these things? There is more than one approach to seeking PTSD therapy. Find the solutions that work best for you, and try more than one therapy approach:

- Stress management
- Anger management
- Assertiveness training
- Couples therapy
- Family Counseling
- Family education courses
- Group therapy
- One-on-one cognitive behavioral therapy

Relationships may seem hazardous if you've endured horrific experiences, but interacting with others in healthy, sustainable ways is incredibly crucial for individuals with PTSD. Everyone needs a support network, and even while forging these sorts of relationships might seem hazardous, social support is a great protective factor for those with PTSD—not to mention those who've endured trauma and are at risk for PTSD.

Strong connections might help you counter some of your emotional responsibilities and ease feelings of isolation and loneliness. As you strive towards better relationships, you may also boost your self-esteem, battling back emotions of guilt, rage, terror, and sadness. In time, you may even be able to reach out to another trauma victim and assist them—a great experience.

Understanding the effects of PTSD

1. **Environmental Triggers**

When a person gets triggered and has an episode such as yelling or pounding drywall, they are typically not conscious that their reaction is due to unresolved trauma. They may look at their environment or the people around them as a cause and blame them.

2. Avoidance

PTSD may cause the individual to feel insensitive and in extreme conditions, may lead to the person's dissociation (i.e. not feeling attached or believing the world is unreal). It is really challenging for a person to remain present at this point with their symptoms.

3. Hypervigilance

This shows up as having to be continually on guard and being unable to relax, which fills the body with stress chemicals, producing physical health difficulties. They may have difficulty with sleeping and attention which might significantly influence their relationships.

4. False Sense Of Reality

A person may look at this world through a warped viewpoint and cling to negative views such as 'The world is unsafe' or 'I am a nasty person'. That may damage their bonds. Negative beliefs end up functioning as self-fulfilling predictions and ruin any connection.

5. Negative Moods

They may reveal unfavorable changes in cognition and emotions that have started or worsened after the stressful occurrence. They cannot remember significant events of a stressful occurrence, which is termed dissociative amnesia. They always have emotions, such as fear, wrath, remorse, or humiliation.

They no longer exhibit interest in formerly fun hobbies, and they may feel alone, detached, or unhappy. Worst of all, they are unable to experience nice feelings like love, tenderness, and happiness.

Chapter 3

Dealing with Triggers

When you deal with PTSD, it frequently seems hard to foresee when an encounter may trigger your symptoms to flare up. However, while it may seem that symptoms emerge out of nowhere, in most instances they are cued by things termed triggers.

PTSD triggers force a person to re-experience a distressing incident.

Traumatic or stressful situations are undesirable and frequent aspects of life. Although a majority of people will encounter some type of trauma in their lives, a tiny number of those people will go on to develop post-traumatic stress disorder (PTSD).

PTSD triggers may vary based on the sort of trauma experienced and might be directly tied to the event, or something unrelated. Examples of PTSD triggers might include persons associated with the traumatic incident, certain items, noises, or locations. For persons who know their triggers, they may go to considerable efforts to avoid them or feel on edge or avoidant if they believe they may face these triggers. PTSD triggers may be frequent among combat veterans, persons with drug use problems, or those exposed to stressful circumstances.

Internal triggers cover the feelings, thoughts, memories, emotions, and physiological sensations that you feel or experience that might trigger the symptoms of PTSD. Internal PTSD triggers could include emotions of worry, irritation, vulnerability, wrath, and/or grief.

External triggers are the people, places, and events that you can meet during your day that might bring back memories of the traumatic experience. External PTSD triggers could include media triggers such as TV programs, movies, and news, seeing persons or qualities of people that remind them of the traumatic incident, or locational signals such as specific buildings or places.

How do triggers develop?

PTSD triggers are generated before or during a traumatic experience, and typically comprise little events or sensations that happened leading up to the catastrophe. For example, someone may hear footsteps or smell smoke leading up to a distressing incident. The brain then identifies a trigger with a future threat or danger; the scent, person, or emotion then functions as a warning signal.

Even if a trigger is not at all linked to a traumatic experience, the brain might build a connection between the two. This connection may lead a person to re-experience their trauma if they encounter that trigger. These encounters are intense, emotional, and maybe anxiety-inducing and debilitating.

Reactions to triggers may emerge in many different ways. For example, triggers may cause:

- Dreams or strong recollections of the horrific incident
- Anxiety or panic attacks
- Aggression or violence
- Extreme sadness
- A heightened startle reaction, or looking "jumpy"
- A desire to "numb the pain" of the tragedy via drug usage

Different Kinds of Triggers

PTSD triggers depend on the sights, sounds, or people that are around a person leading up to or during a traumatic event. Although many people are acutely aware of what triggers them, some people — particularly if they have sensory triggers — may not be sure what causes them to relive their experience.

Triggers are associated with an extreme fear response and can include:

- **People:** People who were near an event that was traumatic, or were perpetrators of trauma can evoke distress
- **Places:** People with PTSD might relive their trauma by revisiting places that are linked to a traumatic event
- **Feelings:** Particular feelings, like worry, panic, or stress, can remind a person of how they felt during a traumatic experience and cause them to relive their experience
- **Things:** Certain objects that were present or implicated in a traumatic experience can trigger an emotional response related to PTSD. This could be a piece of clothing, a type of vehicle, or anything that held significance or was notable leading up to or during the trauma.
- **Scents:** A certain smell, like smoke or a particular aftershave, can also evoke traumatic memories. Scents are thought to have a stronger connection to memory than some of the other senses and may be

linked with an extreme reaction if triggered.
- **Sounds:** Sounds that are the same or similar to a sound that was part of a traumatic event can be extremely triggering. Sound-based triggers are particularly common among war veterans or victims of violent crime.
- **Anniversaries:** Knowing the anniversary or significant dates surrounding a traumatic event can be anxiety-inducing for people with PTSD. The awareness of a significant date can bring on thoughts, feelings, and memories related to trauma.

Identifying and recognizing PTSD triggers

PTSD triggers are not always obvious; someone with PTSD might not be aware of what sets them off or provokes their feelings of fear or anger. This is particularly true with sensory triggers like smells, colors, tastes, or touch.

Recognizing triggers may require a combination of talk therapy, or observation by a psychiatrist to examine parts of the environment that provoke an emotional response.

Recognizing PTSD triggers when they occur can be different for different people. While some people may be fearful or avoidant, others may be angry, aggressive, or panicked. While some people may be able to recognize these behaviors in themselves, others may not. In these cases, healthcare professionals and family and friends may be needed to help to identify triggers.

Coping with PTSD triggers

Although avoiding triggers may seem like a logical way to avoid reliving the trauma, it's unlikely to help with symptoms of PTSD in the long term. Quite the contrary, exposure to triggers is the most common and effective treatment for PTSD. This can help to remove a trigger from the traumatic context and place it in the present, where it doesn't hold any value or association.

People can also cope with PTSD triggers through peer support groups, mindfulness and relaxation strategies, or the assistance of an emotional support animal. In many cases, a combination of personal coping strategies and exposure therapy supported by a psychiatrist can be beneficial.

Posttraumatic Stress Disorder (PTSD) plays a significant role in substance abuse. Often, those who suffer will self-medicate to deal with the symptoms they may experience. Learning to avoid PTSD triggers will help sufferers proactively deal with their past trauma and avoid turning to substances for relief.

Some of the treatment options for managing PTSD triggers include:

Cognitive behavioral therapy (CBT)

Prolonged exposure therapy

Eye movement desensitization and reprocessing (EMDR)

Couples Therapy

Group therapy

Medication

1. Cognitive behavioral therapy (CBT)

CBT is often considered the first line of defense against trauma. Research shows that it can be effective in relieving the symptoms of PTSD.

It works by helping you identify unhelpful thought patterns, learn coping skills to deal with difficult situations, and gain a better understanding of why other people behave the way they do, according to the APA.

There is no set time for how long CBT takes to help you heal from trauma. It can be a few months to several years, depending on progress.

2. Prolonged exposure (PE) therapy

Since most people want to avoid anything that has to do with trauma, this modality teaches you how to gradually confront the feelings associated with a trigger in a safe environment.

PE deals primarily with the avoidance aspect of trauma. The reminders of traumatic experiences that you seek to avoid are faced head-on by repeatedly talking about (and thereby exposing yourself to) the traumatic memories in a safe environment. The purpose is to gain control over your thoughts and feelings so that you can regain your quality of life.

With one session a week, it usually occurs for 3 months. Research shows that this method may be useful for those with chronic, or reoccurring, PTSD.

3. Eye movement desensitization and reprocessing (EMDR)

Unlike other trauma therapies that focus on thought patterns, this method works directly with memory.

After you've chosen what memory or event you'd like to work on, a trained clinician will have you focus on the memory while using a series of soft tones or gentle, alternating taps. As thoughts about the event emerge, you'll have a chance to process them in a new way.

EMDR is an excellent treatment for PTSD. It helps you process trauma and can ease intense reactions to triggers.

EMDR sessions can be scheduled once or twice per week. The total number of sessions varies from between 6 and 12, but some people may not need as many.

Research shows that EMDR is effective for PTSD and can reduce anxiety, depression, and paranoia.

4. Couples Therapy Options

If you and your partner are looking to do therapy together, the most heavily researched and well-known type of couples counseling where one partner has PTSD is cognitive-behavioral conjoint therapy (CBCT). It was uniquely designed to decrease PTSD symptoms and improve relationship adjustment based on a cognitive-behavioral, interpersonal theory of PTSD.

This theory suggests that cognitive, behavioral, and affective processes all work together to affect the individual and their partner such that their interactions serve to maintain PTSD symptoms and relational difficulties.

CBCT looks at themes in your relationship and prioritizes sharing thoughts and feelings. It consists of fifteen 75-minute sessions and aims to make meaning of the traumatic experience.

Other ways to deal with triggers

Another step in dealing with triggers is to identify them. This is done by recognizing when you begin to experience PTSD symptoms. Once this list is compiled you can begin to focus on how to deal with these triggers. Although usually impractical, the best way to cope with triggers is to avoid them altogether. An example of this would be to manage your environment by avoiding certain places that trigger PTSD symptoms.

Unfortunately, it is not possible to avoid all possible triggers. Therefore, it is important to learn various ways of coping with triggers.

So what are some things you can do, in addition to CBT and any other treatments recommended by your doctor, to keep your PTSD symptoms under control? Here are a few approaches you may want to consider.

1. Mindfulness meditation

Increasingly, meditation and mindfulness-based relaxation techniques have been shown to help manage a range of disorders.

Making yourself aware of where you are, in the present moment, and knowing that at that moment you are alright can work to alleviate the anxiety and fear that has been triggered.

A review of mindfulness-based treatments for PTSD points to a few therapies that have been found effective in reducing avoidance and self-blame in people diagnosed with the disorder. These are:

- mindfulness-based stress reduction (MBSR), which is an intensive 8-week program focused on the practice of mindfulness meditation that aims to train people to focus their attention on their breath and learn to avoid getting carried away by intrusive thoughts
- mindfulness-based cognitive therapy (MBCT), defined as "an adaptation of MBSR," has a very similar structure but is

designed to target depressive moods and negative thoughts, more specifically
- mindfulness-based exposure therapy, which includes a 16-week non-trauma-focused program that incorporates MBCT techniques and favors safe and controlled exposure to avoided stimuli, focusing on self-compassion training
- meditation-relaxation, such as loving-kindness meditation, was also deemed effective in increasing self-compassion and reducing depressive symptoms related to PTSD, mantra repetition practice, which refers to "the silent repeating of a sacred word or phrase," appears to be effective in targeting anger, hyperarousal, or the state of being constantly on guard, and symptoms of anxiety and depression

2. Regain focus via physical activity

Many individuals who have been diagnosed with PTSD claim that finding an engaging physical activity that they can undertake frequently has helped them to lessen their levels of stress and live with their symptoms.

Researchers from Anglia Ruskin University in Cambridge in the United Kingdom showed that surfing may be an excellent coping mechanism for combat veterans diagnosed with PTSD.

According to the team, this sport assists veterans to enter a concentrated mental state known as "flow," in which they are so immersed in the action they are practicing that all other thoughts and emotions are pushed away.

Dr. Nick Caddick, who was engaged in the research, equates this with the benefits of mindfulness meditation, simply that it is more active. He calls it "a moving type of mindfulness."

Medical News Today also reported on research that claimed that Tai chi — a kind of martial art — might aid military veterans to control their PTSD symptoms.

3. Aromatherapy

Another research published by MNT indicated that orange essential oil may be useful in lowering symptoms of chronic stress and anxiety linked with PTSD. However, this research was only done in mice, and these results have yet to be reproduced in a human cohort.

Some claim that aromatherapy might be useful in controlling chronic stress.

Still, some persons diagnosed with PTSD have indicated that aromatherapy may be a beneficial relaxing method and is good at decreasing stress levels.

Sezin Koehler — who has been treating her PTSD symptoms for many years — adds, "Lavender, sage, peppermint, or any other soothing oil applied on the region between your eyebrows and your pulse points is beautifully calming."

Author and former Thames Valley Police officer David Kinchin, who was diagnosed with PTSD in the 1990s, also argues for the calming impact of aromatherapy in one of his books.

"Aromatherapy may form part of a treatment routine as well as being a preventative therapy in its own right. It delivers pleasure via the sense of touch (massage), the sense of smell (aromatic oils), and the sense of sight (pleasant surroundings) [...] By thus so, it helps to establish favorable circumstances in body and mind for healing to take place fairly naturally."

-David Kinchin, 'Post Traumatic Stress Disorder: The Invisible Injury'.

4. Art therapy

A sort of PTSD treatment that has been building up pace over the last several years is art therapy.

Led by professionals trained to deal with people who have encountered traumatic experiences, this style of therapy tries to help individuals externalize their feelings and learn to cope with difficult memories via art, such as painting or sculpture.

One case study reveals how art therapy may enable patients diagnosed with PTSD and traumatic brain injury to overcome their symptoms and begin to put their upsetting experiences behind them by utilizing art projects wisely.

Study author Melissa Walker, who works as an art therapist, addressed why and how art therapy may be successful in treating PTSD in a dedicated TED talk.

Walker invites the individuals that she works with to construct masks examining the influence of the horrific incidents on their lives and personalities.

"Someone who has suffered trauma has a barrier that inhibits them from verbalizing what they've gone through," she adds in an interview. "There is a shutdown in the [convolution of] Broca —

the region of the brain responsible for speech and language."

"The mask provides them an opportunity to explain themselves. The solid picture of the mask releases words. It reintegrates the left and right hemispheres. Now they may address their emotions with their social worker or psychiatrist."

5. Pets for PTSD

Another option allegedly beneficial in helping individuals to deal with the disruptive symptoms of PTSD is adopting a pet that is carefully taught to identify and avoid — or stop — the beginning of such symptoms.

Several studies have indicated that adopting a trained animal has a beneficial effect, at least in the short-term, by helping patients to manage PTSD-related despair and anxiety, as well as other symptoms such as nightmares.

A study found that spending as little as 1 week with a professionally trained dog decreased PTSD symptoms by 82 percent.

Richard Steinberg, a soldier diagnosed with PTSD, claims that his dog "can detect when [he's] having a nightmare, night sweats," and she gets restless, doing her best to capture his attention, "trying to remove [him] from the situation."

"Putting my hands on her calms me down, and it calms her down," he says. "She notices the chemical changes in my body."

6. Using your recovery support system

Talking to someone who understands your PTSD and is helpful in your recovery, is a method to let go of the effects of being triggered.

7. Telling yourself the truth

Identifying that the sensation or scenario you are in is not the same as your traumatic incident, and being aware that your dread and anxiety, although genuine, are not always realistic responses. Remind yourself that you are secure now. Positive self-talk or writing when provoked feelings come up might be useful in coping with such emotions.

8. Using grounding methods

Grounding techniques utilize your senses to return to the present moment, much like mindfulness. Grasp a particular item, listen to music, smell or taste something with a strong aroma or flavor, take note of your surroundings, or hold someone's hand to bring yourself back into the here and now.

Dealing with PTSD triggers in recovery isn't easy, but with awareness and some practice, it may become a lot more bearable.

Other methods include:
- Deep breathing exercises
- Yoga

- Expressive writing
- Acupuncture
- Gradual relaxation methods

Along with complimentary treatments, consider keeping a balanced lifestyle.

If you can, obtain between 7 and 9 hours of excellent sleep per night and consider eating a diet that comprises enough nutrient-dense foods.

When feasible, it may be a good idea to spare some time for relaxation methods and interacting with your loved ones regularly.

The more coping methods you acquire, the more effective you will be in controlling your triggers. And by properly managing PTSD triggers you will be less likely to develop harmful coping techniques, such as drug misuse.

Negative coping mechanisms may appear useful on the spur of the moment, although they may quickly become self-destructive in the long term. These may include succumbing to alcohol or recreational drugs to dull your emotions, alleviate tension, or quieten your thoughts.

Alcohol and other drugs may take the edge off in the beginning. However, they might induce addiction if used as a replacement for a suitable treatment, such as cognitive behavioral therapy (CBT), which has been acknowledged as a "safe and effective intervention" for this illness.

Chapter 4

Help and Support for Your Loved One

When a spouse, friend, or a family member suffers post-traumatic stress disorder (PTSD) it affects you, too. PTSD isn't easy to live with and it may take a significant toll on relationships and family life.

You may be wounded by your loved one's remoteness and moodiness or straining to comprehend their behavior—why they are less loving and more volatile. You may feel like you're walking on eggshells or living with a stranger. You may also have to take up a higher share of domestic responsibilities and cope with the frustration of a loved one who won't open up. The symptoms of PTSD may even lead to job loss, drug misuse, and other issues that impact the entire family.

It's hard not to take the symptoms of PTSD personally, but it's crucial to understand that a person with PTSD may not always have control over their conduct. Your loved one's nervous system is "stuck" in a state of perpetual alert, making them repeatedly feel vulnerable and dangerous, or having to relive the horrific incident again and over. This may lead to anger, impatience, despair, distrust, and other PTSD symptoms that your loved one can't simply choose to turn off.

With the correct assistance from you and other family and friends, however, your loved one's nervous system may get "unstuck." With these recommendations, you may assist them to ultimately move on from the horrific experience and allow your life together to return to normal.

When someone you care about suffers from post-traumatic stress disorder, it may be stressful. But with these actions, you can assist your loved one go on with their life.

Helping someone with PTSD

Tip 1: Provide social support

It's normal for persons with PTSD to withdraw from family and friends. They may feel humiliated, not want to burden others or assume that other people won't understand what they're going through. While it's crucial to respect your loved one's limits, your comfort and support may help them overcome emotions of helplessness, loss, and despair. Trauma specialists feel that face-to-face support from others is the most critical aspect of PTSD rehabilitation.

Knowing how to effectively display your love and support for someone with PTSD isn't always simple. You can't force your loved one to get well, but you can play a huge part in the healing process by just spending time with them.

Don't push your loved one into talking. It may be quite difficult for those with PTSD to speak about their horrific experiences. For others, it might even make them feel worse. Instead, let them know you're ready to listen when they want to chat, or simply hang around when they don't. Comfort for someone with PTSD comes from feeling involved and accepted by you, not necessarily from chatting.

Do "normal" activities with your loved one, things that have nothing to do with PTSD or the terrible incident. Encourage your loved one to seek out companions, explore activities that offer them joy, and engage in rhythmic activities such as walking, jogging, swimming, or rock climbing. Take a fitness class together, go dancing, or establish a regular lunch appointment with friends and family.

Let your loved one take the lead, rather than instructing them what to do. Everyone with PTSD is different yet most individuals intuitively know what helps them feel peaceful and comfortable. Take clues from your loved one as to how you might best give support and company.

Tip 2: Be a good listener

While you shouldn't encourage a person with PTSD to communicate if they do want to share, try to listen without expectations or judgments. Make it evident that you're interested and that you care, but don't stress about delivering advice. It's the act of listening carefully that is useful to your loved one, not what you say.

A person with PTSD may need to speak about the painful incident over and over again. This is part of the healing process, so resist the desire to advise your loved one to stop reliving the past and move on. Instead, offer to chat as many times as they need.

Some of the things your loved one says could be quite hard to listen to. It's alright to detest what you hear, but it's crucial to respect their sentiments and responses. If you come across as disapproving, terrified, or critical, they are unlikely to open up to you again.

Tip 3: Rebuild trust and safety

Trauma transforms the way a person perceives the world, making it appear like a continuously hazardous and terrifying place. It also impairs people's capacity to trust others and themselves. If there's any way you can recreate your loved one's feeling of security, it will help their rehabilitation.

Express your dedication to the relationship. Let your loved one know that you're here for the long haul so they feel cherished and supported.

Create routines. Structure and consistent routines help provide a feeling of stability and comfort to those with PTSD, including adults and children. Creating routines might mean asking your loved one to assist with shopping or housekeeping, for example, maintaining regular times for meals, or just "being there" for the individual.

Minimize stress at home. Try to make sure your loved one gets space and time for relaxation.

Speak about the future and establish preparations. This may help combat the prevalent sensation among persons with PTSD that their future is restricted.

Keep your commitments. Help reestablish trust by proving that you're trustworthy. Be consistent and follow through on what you claim you're going to do.

Emphasize your loved one's strengths. Tell your loved one you feel they're capable of rehabilitation and point out all of their excellent characteristics and triumphs.

Look for strategies to empower your loved one. Rather than doing things for them that they're capable of doing for themselves, it's preferable to increase their confidence and self-trust by providing them with more options and control.

Tip 4: Anticipate and control triggers

A trigger is anything—a person, place, object, or situation—that reminds your loved one of the trauma and triggers a PTSD symptom, such as a flashback. Sometimes, triggers are evident. For example, a military veteran could be triggered by seeing his warmates or by the loud sounds that seem like firing.

Others may take some time to recognize and comprehend, such as hearing a song that was playing while the traumatic incident occurred, so that song or even others in the same musical genre are triggers.

Similarly, triggers don't have to be external. Internal sentiments and sensations might potentially provoke PTSD symptoms.

Common external PTSD triggers include:

- Sights, sounds, or odors connected with the trauma.
- People, places, or things that evoke trauma.
- Significant dates or periods, such as anniversaries or a certain time of day.

- Nature (various sorts of weather, seasons, etc). (certain types of weather, seasons, etc.).
- Conversations or media coverage concerning trauma or unpleasant news occurrences.
- Situations that seem restricting (stuck in traffic, at the doctor's office, in a throng).
- Relationship, family, school, job, or money demands or disputes.
- Funerals, hospitals, or medical care.

Common internal PTSD triggers include:

- Physical discomfort, such as hunger, thirst, exhaustion, illness, and sexual dissatisfaction.
- Any bodily evidence that's a reminder to the event, including pain, previous wounds, scars, or a comparable injury.
- Strong feelings, particularly feeling powerless, out of control, or imprisoned.
- Sentiments toward family members include contradictory feelings of affection, vulnerability, and hatred.

Talking to your loved one about PTSD triggers

Ask your loved one about things they've done in the past to react to a trigger that appeared to help (as well as the ones that didn't). Then come up with a collaborative game plan for how you will react in the future.

Decide with your loved one how you should react when they suffer a nightmare, flashback, or panic attack. Having a strategy in place will make the situation less terrifying for both of you. You'll also be in a far better position to assist your loved one calm down.

How to assist someone experiencing a flashback or panic attack

During a flashback, individuals typically have a sensation of disassociation, as if they're absent from their bodies. Anything you can do to "ground" them will assist.

Tell your loved one they're experiencing a flashback and that even though it seems genuine, the incident is not truly occurring again.

Help remind them of their surroundings (for example, encourage them to glance around the room and explain out loud what they observe).

Encourage them to take deep, steady breaths (hyperventilating can intensify feelings of panic).

Avoid rapid movements or anything that can shock them.

Ask before you touch them. Touching or placing your arms around the individual could make them feel imprisoned, which can lead to increased irritation and even violence.

Tip 5: Deal with instability and wrath

PTSD may lead to difficulty controlling emotions and impulses. In your loved one, this may emerge as severe irritation, moodiness, or eruptions of fury.

People suffering from PTSD live in a perpetual state of physical and mental stress. Since they frequently have difficulties sleeping, it means they're continuously weary, on edge, and physically strung out—increasing the probability that they'll overreact to day-to-day pressures.

For many persons with PTSD, rage may also be a cover for other emotions such as loss, helplessness, or guilt. Anger makes people feel strong, instead of weak and defenseless. Others strive to conceal their wrath until it emerges when you least expect it.

Watch for signals that your loved one is furious, such as tightening jaws or fists, talking loudly, or growing impatient. Take action to defuse the situation as soon as you observe the earliest warning indicators.

Try to stay calm. During an emotional outburst, do your best to keep cool. This will indicate to your loved one that you are "safe," and avoid the issue from escalating.

Give the individual room. Avoid crowding or grasping the individual. This might make a traumatized person feel threatened.

Ask how you can assist. For example: "What can I do to assist you right now?" You may also propose a time out or change of scenery.

Put safety first. If the individual grows more furious despite your efforts to calm him or her down, leave the home or lock yourself in a room. Call the police if you worry that your loved one may injure himself or others.

Help your loved one regulate their rage. Rage is a natural, healthy emotion, but when persistent, explosive anger spirals out of control, it may have major implications for a person's relationships, health, and state of mind. Your loved one may bring anger under control by understanding the fundamental causes and adopting better methods to express their frustrations.

Tip 6: Support Therapy

Despite the value of your love and support, it isn't always enough. Many individuals who have been traumatized require expert PTSD counseling. But bringing it up might be uncomfortable. Think about how you'd feel if someone advised that you required treatment.

Wait for the proper moment to share your concerns. Don't bring it up while you're bickering or in the thick of a crisis. Also, be cautious with your terminology. Avoid anything that indicates that your loved one is "crazy." Frame it in a positive, practical light: therapy is a chance to gain new skills that can be utilized to address a broad range of PTSD-related issues.

Emphasize the positives. For example, treatment may help kids become more autonomous and in charge. Or it can assist minimize the anxiety and avoidance that is stopping them from accomplishing the things they wish to do.

Focus on particular issues. If your loved one closes down when you speak about PTSD or therapy, concentrate instead on how treatment may assist with particular difficulties like anger management, anxiety, or attention and memory problems.

Acknowledge the inconveniences and limits of treatment. For example, you may remark, "I realize that counseling isn't a fast or miraculous solution, and it may take a time to locate the perfect therapist. But even if it helps a little, it will be worth it."

Enlist aid from those your loved one respects and trusts. The individual with PTSD may be more amenable to therapy if the suggestion comes from someone else. Suggest the individual consult a doctor or chat with a specific friend, teacher, coach, or religious leader, for example.

Encourage your loved one to join a support group. Getting associated with others who have gone through similar horrific events might help some persons with PTSD feel less damaged and alone.

More ways to help your loved one

1. Learn what makes your spouse feel secure

Fear is a fundamental characteristic of PTSD, according to a study. One technique to prevent fear is by establishing a safe atmosphere.

One of the things that partners can truly do to help their loved ones with PTSD is merely to discover what might make them feel comfortable.

When your spouse or friend is feeling uncomfortable, you could consider doing what will assist them experience a sense of security or comfort depending on how they feel most loved and secure, such as:

- extending an embrace
- delivering vocal affirmations, such as "it's going to be OK"
- cooking for them, or giving them a modest gift
- spending additional quality time together

There's one catch, though: When offering this protection, make sure you aren't deliberately assisting your loved one to avoid what they dread. One example of this would be constantly traveling an out-of-the-way path to avoid the site of an automobile accident to make your spouse feel secure.

The greatest thing you can do for your loved one is let them determine when they're ready to engage with something and support them in their decision-making.

2. Reassure them

Reassuring your loved one of their value and lovability is one easy yet effective technique to help someone with PTSD.

When Foo was in the depths of complicated PTSD, her buddy whispered five words she'll never forget: "You are easy to love." She told Psych Central she found relief in both the substance of her friend's statements and their recurrence over time. You are simple to adore.

These were soothing words for Foo. What words of encouragement do your partner or friend find comforting?

Some examples may include personalized variants of the following:

- "I am not going anywhere."
- "You will get through this."
- "I love you."
- "We're in this together. I'm on your side no matter what."
- "Please know I'm here for you."

Someone dealing with PTSD may perceive reminders of prior trauma even if there's nothing external that supports a sense of risk. During these times, particular verbal reassurance from a loved one may help balance panic and bring in a feeling of peace.

3. Stay in clear communication

Each individual will have distinct symptoms and causes. Clear communication may help you prepare the most helpful ways to react when they emerge. Communicating about symptoms and triggers may allow you to establish a deliberate, supportive response.

For example, one typical symptom of PTSD and complicated PTSD is dissociation. If your spouse or acquaintance has dissociation, they may demonstrate a feeling of numbness or detachment.

If your loved one begins conversing with you with a flat voice, or flat affect, it may be first hard to decipher. It's good to ask questions about what their expression or tone may or may not convey.

One way you may help your spouse is by telling them, "Hey, you seem sort of annoyed. What are you feeling right now? Is there anything I can do?"

If you and your loved one have formed a rapport regarding symptoms, you may feel safe asking them directly about what a blank look may signify. If you're still learning about how PTSD presents for your loved one, it may take time to find out what your communication style will be.

In any situation, it helps to be in regular touch regarding both parties' wants and expectations to demonstrate love and prevent misinterpretation.

4. Do some grounding exercises together

When triggers happen, there are a few evidence-based ways that individuals with PTSD may take to control their nervous system and feel more grounded or present. You may offer to sit with your loved one and conduct some of these techniques together. In doing so, you may find yourself feeling more peaceful and present, too.

Over time, regulating activities with a loved one — known as co-regulation — may help your loved one control their nervous system. It may also make you and your spouse feel more at ease and connected.

5. Affirm their strengths

While it's vital not to celebrate the qualities one creates out of trauma, it may be useful to recognize, validate, and appreciate the ways someone with PTSD has evolved during their recovery path.

Identifying and affirming strengths may sound like the following:

- "I applaud your bravery."
- "I applaud your skill to cope."
- "I've observed how powerful you are. Do you (or can you) recognize your strength?"

Foo believes that her recovery path with complex PTSD has "allowed me to feel less like, 'I'm a terrible person who can't do anything right' and more like, 'You know, I have a condition that sometimes takes a little more care, but it doesn't make me a horrible person.'"

Creating Emotional Safety

Understanding how to build emotional safety is crucial to creating meaningful connections and successful relationships.

Emotional safety is the cornerstone of a loving and healthy relationship. It's about creating trust with another person and feeling secure enough, to be honest, and vulnerable with them.

To put it simply, emotional safety is feeling confident enough to genuinely express yourself with someone and show up as your most honest self.

Emotional safety also goes both ways. When you feel emotionally secure and disclose your genuine self, it opens the door for your spouse to do the same. And when both individuals in a relationship feel comfortable, it offers a safe setting where a deeper and more loving connection may grow.

Emotional safety does not apply to violent relationships. If you're facing abuse, whether physical or emotional, you have various alternatives for obtaining assistance. Try reaching out to a trustworthy friend, family member, or therapist or phoning a domestic abuse hotline.

What are the advantages of an emotionally safe relationship?

When you find yourself in an emotionally secure relationship, odds are you'll enjoy several perks as a consequence. Benefits of emotionally secure partnerships include:

- You feel respected and valuable.
- You may fully be yourself without the worry of condemnation.

- You may exhibit your shortcomings without being taken advantage of.
- You may share fearlessly and express yourself freely.
- You feel seen, heard, and understood.
- More significantly, an emotionally secure relationship fosters a stronger bond.

Of connection, Brené Brown, author and research professor of social work at the University of Houston, said it best: "I define connection as the energy that exists between people when they feel seen, heard, and valued; when they can give and receive without judgment; and when they derive sustenance and strength from the relationship."

Ways to promote emotional safety in your relationship

Wondering how to establish emotional safety or uncertain about where to start? Here are some useful methods to foster trust and vulnerability in every relationship.

1. Respect boundaries and consent

Setting and maintaining boundaries may promote safety and security in a relationship by defining personal limitations. By stating a constraint, you let your spouse in on your preferences and ask them to share their own. Think of limits as not just defending yourself but also safeguarding your connection.

Boundaries might be physical, sexual, intellectual, emotional, or financial – all crucial to developing respect in a healthy partnership. Once you create a boundary, you and your partner must respect it. Some examples of boundaries that enhance emotional safety are:

- recognizing what is essential to you
- sharing personal information gradually
- protecting your time by not overcommitting

- asking for space when you need alone time
- conveying your comfort level on intimacy

2. Pay attention to your nonverbal communication

Body language is vital for emotional safety. Vocal tone, eye shape, posture, and other micro expressions are continually being interpreted by you and your partner, whether you recognize it or not.

"If you approach your partners with a hard gaze, tightly squeezed lips, and brief phrases, they may not feel safe," says Dr. Jake Porter, a Houston-based certified professional counselor.

"The important thing here is to remember that we are individually accountable not just for the things we speak but also the method we communicate them," he says.

It's a good idea to practice paying attention to the nonverbal signals you're carrying with you before you approach your partner. Consider asking yourself, "What is my body language sending right now?"

3. Be an engaged listener

Active listening is a vital component of a good relationship because individuals need to be heard and understood to feel comfortable and valued. "Active listening is when you lay aside your barriers and distractions, and fully take in what your partner is telling you," says Dr. Isabelle Morley, a certified clinical psychologist located in Massachusetts.

"The capacity to actively listen implies that anytime anxieties or problems occur, your spouse will feel safe telling you," she says. "Instead of the situation escalating or your spouse feeling resentful, you'll be able to swiftly and simply handle it."

Some strategies to practice active listening include:

- nonverbal indications of listening including smiling, nodding, and keeping eye contact
- asking your partner questions or asking for clarification

4. Practice transparency

Transparency is a vital aspect of creating trust and emotional safety. When you practice transparency, you avoid the possible sensation that you or your spouse are concealing anything from one another.

While you don't need to disclose every area of your life with your spouse, "general openness about your ideas, emotions, and activities is a wonderful approach to create trust, communication, and security," adds Morley.

5. Give your spouse the benefit of the doubt

Giving your spouse the benefit of the doubt entails eliminating judgment and, instead, being inquisitive to learn about the rationale for their conduct. Most people's motives are subconscious and frequently tied to the personal baggage they bring to the relationship.

When we stop criticizing and making up tales about why our spouses did what they did, we begin to look at them positively from a position of compassion and understanding. We may disagree with them, but we can at least provide a secure atmosphere without conflict.

6. Foster responsibility and follow through

Following through tells your spouse that you are reliable and appreciate the connection. When you commit to something and follow through, you actively establish trust by showing your spouse your dedication. Yet following through doesn't have to happen immediately.

Even when you take tiny efforts, allowing your spouse to see your persistent effort shows them your devotion to the connection. Try keeping your spouse in the loop, since this will help you hold yourself responsible too.

7. Consider couples or relationship counseling

A mental health professional's viewpoint may assist individuals in relationships to create emotional safety by concentrating on coping with conflict rather than focusing on the problem itself.

Couples counseling develops emotional safety by helping couples understand how they function together as a system. The treatment is less focused on the content the couples are arguing over and more on the process of how they argue.

Focusing on the content could assist them at the moment but they are simply going to wind right back in the therapy office next time they can't agree. Instead, helping them establish a new process for how they address conflict will set them up for success as life continues to throw hurdles their way.

Chapter 5

Communicating with Your Loved One

Communicating the appropriate approach is highly crucial when supporting a loved one with PTSD. Remember that good language empowers.

When writing or speaking about persons with disabilities or combat-related injuries, it is crucial to put the person first. Group designations such as "the blind," "the retarded" or "the handicapped" are improper since they do not represent the uniqueness, equality, or dignity of persons with disabilities. Further, phrases like "normal person" indicate that the person with a handicap isn't normal, but "person without a disability" is descriptive but not negative.

Here are methods that'll strengthen your communication with your loved one

1. Listen without any hidden motives

People are typically programmed to listen with other purposes in mind, whether it's to convince, judge, or create an impression, we often listen for self-serving reasons. How frequently do we listen, simply for the purpose of listening?

Loved ones who have PTSD are sensitive to our intentions because of what they're experiencing. In their thoughts, individuals may feel as if no one can grasp what is going on in their brains and that others simply want to overwhelm them with harmful counsel.

One of the most effective methods to connect with someone suffering from trauma is simply listening for the sake of it: listening to comprehend, empathize, and record what your loved one is feeling. By listening without hidden agendas, you offer doors for others to be vulnerable and receptive to obtaining aid.

2. Ask how you can assist with triggers

Once individuals have opened up about their thoughts and emotions, it may also be good to inquire about handling triggers.

PTSD may be triggered by particular triggers, such as an event that's comparable to trauma-causing events, a sight, sound, scent, or other things. It might be of great assistance if you ask folks how you can aid in handling these stressors.

Sometimes, it's not only avoiding triggers but assisting individuals to deal with and react to unexpected events. Other methods you may offer your support through hardships and triggers include:

- Expressing that you're available to listen.
- Reminding him or her of prospective circumstances where they may encounter triggers.
- Telling him or her ahead of time whether a trigger may arise.

- Helping him or her discover strategies to relax in circumstances that may be leading to flashbacks or other signs of stress.

Being attentive to your loved one's triggers might positively improve how they live with PTSD.

3. Give them alternatives to start obtaining assistance

As much as possible, you don't want to coerce individuals into obtaining treatment. Treating a dual diagnosis, or a disease that involves a mental illness such as PTSD, as well as an issue with alcohol or drugs, is simpler and more successful when patients have the drive to do so.

If you have a loved one who is hesitant about obtaining aid, don't impose your views straight immediately. Instead, you may give choices and explain how each one might assist. Give individuals the right to pick what they believe may work for them, such as obtaining therapy, going to rehab, or having a medical checkup beforehand.

Allowing the space and flexibility to choose may enable your loved ones to feel in control of their actions, opening the door to self-motivation.

4. Notice and celebrate the minor and major wins.

It's one thing to celebrate your loved one finally stopping drinking or finding a job after rehab–these are amazing successes. However, it may be extremely useful to also highlight their minor triumphs, such as spending more time socializing with others, outside their comfort zones, or managing a difficult circumstance successfully.

Expressing to them that they're on the right road and showing them that you notice them and their successes are methods you may sincerely elevate your loved one, helping them manage PTSD.

5. Understand your involvement in the PTSD struggle

Family and loved ones may take delight in helping and encouraging those with PTSD. While handling PTSD may be tough, employing a few tactics can take your loved one a step closer to recovery.

Additional tips for communicating with people with PTSD

- Stress may occasionally impair a person's conduct or professional performance. Do your best to minimize high-pressure situations.
- People experience trauma differently and will have their own distinct coping and healing strategies, so treat each person as an individual. Ask what will make him or her most comfortable and respect his or her requirements.
- Be patient if the individual repeats his or her tales and experiences, and avoid interrupting the person.

- In a crisis, keep cool, be helpful and remember that the effects of PTSD are natural responses to an abnormal environment.
- Ask how you can assist the individual, and find out if there is a support person you can contact (such as a family member or your company's Employee Assistance Program).
- When appropriate, you can inquire if the individual has medicine that he or she needs to take.
- Remember to relax.
- Treat the person with decency, respect, and kindness.
- Listen to the person.
- Offer help but do not push or be upset if your offer is not accepted.
- Don't be scared to say "I don't know," or "Let me check." You may be open about the boundaries of your power or capacity to react to a person's demands or requests.
- Be careful that symptoms of PTSD may change and are impacted by numerous

things - there may be moments of ease and comfort as well as more stressful times.
- Support, patience, and understanding go a long way. Be generous with them.

Communication hazards to avoid

Don't:

- Give simple answers or carelessly convince your loved one everything is going to be alright.
- Stop your loved one from talking about their emotions or anxieties.
- Offer unsolicited advice or tell your loved one what they "should" do.
- Blame all of your relationship or family troubles on your loved one's PTSD.
- Invalidate, diminish, or reject your loved one's horrific experience.
- Give ultimatums or make threats or demands.

- Make your loved one feel weak because they aren't dealing as well as others.
- Tell your loved one they were fortunate it wasn't worse.
- Take over with your own unique experiences or sentiments.

Chapter 6

Taking Care of Yourself

When you're caring for someone with complex PTSD, their anguish may rapidly become your distress if you don't keep perspective and boundaries and if you don't have enough support yourself.

Yes, taking care of yourself guarantees that you are in the greatest position to care for your loved one, but it's crucial to take care of yourself for your own reason. And only in this manner can you provide an example for your loved one of how to practice committed compassion and self-care.

When someone you love lives with PTSD, their symptoms may also impair your mental health and well-being.

The first thing you can do is to recognize the ailment and its symptoms, so you know what to anticipate.

Managing symptoms of PTSD is feasible, so you don't have to feel trapped. For you, being aware of how the disorder could affect you and your relationship might be useful.

It might be distressing to witness someone you love acting differently. Having an emotional response to what your loved one is going through is both typical and natural.

You could experience:

- fear and worry
- avoidance
- guilt and shame
- anger
- negativity
- health problems
- sleep troubles

1. Fear and worry

If you live with someone who has PTSD, you can be at the receiving end of some of their grief and fury.

You may feel neglected at times, or you might be astonished by your loved one's furious outbursts. As a consequence, you could feel like you're "walking on eggshells."

Someone with PTSD may look unpredictable, particularly if this is new. This might put you on your alert and make home life stressful.

In other situations, you might acquire worry about the unexpected, which to some individuals can be distressing.

2. Avoidance

If your loved one has unpredictable responses, you can be extremely attentive and cautious about upsetting them.

You may start avoiding them or cease talking about particular subjects.

3. Guilt and shame

There are various reasons why you could start experiencing guilt or shame when your loved one has PTSD.

You may feel that there was something you could have done to avoid the trauma, or even feel guilty for your own health and happiness.

You may choose to distance yourself from others as a method to encourage your loved one who isn't ready to mingle. But this might make you feel dissatisfied or angry after a time, which can also bring up guilt.

These are normal and reasonable sentiments, but not necessarily true.

You deserve to be well, just like your loved one — but while you can't alter what happened to them, you can care for them and yourself using services that are accessible to you.

4. Anger

Anger may come on for various reasons. You may have to take on extra domestic or family tasks now. Or you're presented with a new predicament of having to care for your loved one.

It's fairly typical to feel overwhelmed and undervalued when this occurs.

Anger may also be a normal reaction to verbal or violent outbursts, or if your loved one has acquired any drug use concerns.

5. Negativity

Your loved one may not appear like the person you know before PTSD. This could make it challenging to retain the same degree of concern or connection you formerly had.

In certain circumstances, you could feel animosity toward them because they suddenly lack the attributes you valued.

On the other hand, watching your loved one in agony and being exposed to unfamiliar conditions could also place a negative tint on how you perceive the world.

6. Health difficulties

Seeing someone you love suffer may be unpleasant and frustrating for you, too. Chronic stress may then lead to health concerns. Or maybe altered your diet and exercise habits, or you've resorted to drugs like cigarettes or alcohol to cope.

Chronic stress may lead to health concerns, including:

- stomach troubles
- headaches
- muscle pain
- headaches
- Sleep troubles

Sleep disorders may arise from any variety of causes, including the chronic stress indicated above.

You may also be low on sleep as a consequence of your partner's sleeplessness or feel alienated since you have to sleep in different beds. If you're anxious or stressed about your relationship, you may lay awake fretting.

When these challenges become repeated, you can develop a chronic sleep disorder..

Just remember: Taking care of yourself is as vital as delivering assistance to your loved one.

Safeguard your physical, mental, emotional, and spiritual needs. If you are not getting enough sleep, eating healthy, exercising, or doing the activities that you used to like doing, it may be time to seek some family or professional help. You may find occasional relief and establish a crucial and powerful support structure for yourself in the process.

Meanwhile, as you practice excellent listening and create a better understanding of your loved one's feelings, you may be sensitive to your own experiences and required limits.

Draw a line at taking personally what your loved one is going through and how they are expressing it. Take responsibility for your own experience and for being a sensitive and compassionate advocate

Caretakers in relationships with persons with PTSD frequently neglect to take care of themselves. When caring for someone with PTSD will have to be strong a lot of the time. To achieve this, you must take care of your own mental health.

Helping a spouse deal with PTSD is a rehabilitation process that demands patience. The more you take care of yourself, the better you'll be able to aid your spouse with their rehabilitation. Understand that you may still become upset and disappointed, but know that experiencing bad sentiments will pass, and it doesn't diminish your love for them.

While it's crucial to discover how you can help your partner with PTSD, it's equally important to make sure you're taking care of yourself, too.

It's acceptable for you to feel worried, too, while helping your spouse. So make sure you're also getting the alone time you need and are doing activities you like.

Try to remain consistent. Nobody is expecting you to be 'on it' all the time – you'll need rest and leisure too – but try to keep your support consistent, rather than making a tremendous effort when you can see they're suffering, then backing off when it looks like they're doing alright.

Get to know their triggers and truly think about how your secure, home setting may reflect this. For example, if speaking of a specific occurrence or area triggers them, be cautious of what's on TV, or in newspapers, you could leave lying about.

Express your dedication to the relationship. Let the individual know you're here for the long run, no matter what their PTSD may bring.

Create and stay to routines. Structure and regular routines might boost the person's emotions of security. If things need to change, give them as much notice as possible.

Speak about the future and establish preparations. This may help combat the prevalent sensation among persons with PTSD that their future is restricted.

Keep your commitments. Help reestablish trust by being trustworthy. Be consistent and follow through on the things you claim you're going to do.

Tell them you feel they are capable of healing. Help empower them, and accentuate their qualities

More take away

Letting your family member's PTSD rule your life while disregarding your own needs is a guaranteed recipe for exhaustion and may even lead to additional traumatization. You might acquire your own trauma symptoms through listening to trauma tales or being exposed to unsettling symptoms like flashbacks. The more tired and stressed you feel, the higher the danger is that you'll get traumatized.

In order to have the fortitude to be there for your loved one over the long run and minimize your risk for secondary traumatization, you have to nurture and care for yourself.

- Take care of your bodily needs: get adequate sleep, exercise frequently, eat correctly, and look after any medical difficulties.
- Manage your stress. The more calm, peaceful, and concentrated you are, the more you'll be able to aid your loved one.
- Cultivate your own support system. Lean on other family members, trustworthy friends, your own therapist or support group, or your religious community. Talking about your emotions and what

you're going through may be quite therapeutic.
- Make time for your own life. Don't give up friends, hobbies, or things that make you happy. It's crucial to have things in your life that you look forward to.
- Spread the responsibilities. Ask other family members and friends for help so you may take a break. You may also wish to seek out respite options in your neighborhood.
- Set limits. Be realistic about what you're capable of delivering. Know your limitations, convey them to your family members and those concerned, and stick to them.
- Seek therapy. Consider your own mental health.
- Be patient. Recovery is a process that takes time and frequently entails setbacks. The crucial thing is to keep cheerful and continue to support your loved one.
- Educate yourself on PTSD. The more you know about the symptoms, effects, and

treatment choices, the better prepared you'll be to aid your loved one, comprehend what they are going through, and keep things in perspective.

Accept (and anticipate) mixed sentiments. As you go through the emotional wringer, be prepared for a confusing combination of feelings—some of which you'll never want to accept. Just remember, having unfavorable thoughts about your family member doesn't imply you don't love them.

Supporting the ones we love might be some of the most essential and fulfilling jobs we perform.

People with PTSD may depend on loved ones for help. Your actions — from listening to your loved one to expressing that you love them — have the potential to be tremendously useful to your loved one throughout their recovery path.

Manufactured by Amazon.ca
Bolton, ON

35448555R00074